Answers for Ar `GW01417533`

Part 1 - "Do vaccines work?"

Rivelino Montenegro, Ph.D.

If you want a printed copy of this book, you can order by Amazon:

https://www.amazon.com/~/e/B00FCRGAIC

Twitter: @DrRivelino

February 2021

Contents

Do vaccines work?

Science is constantly evolving. What was true yesterday could no longer be valid today. As Sir Arthur Lewis said, "science throws off old skin as it grows." This is even more evident in medicine. There are loads of abandoned theories and treatments. However, there are thousands of other things in medicine that are crystal clear and proven to hold true! One of them is the idea that immunization works.

In countries with high vaccine programme coverage, many of the diseases that were previously responsible for the majority of childhood deaths have essentially disappeared.[1]

The World Health Organization (WHO) estimates that 2–3 million lives are saved each year by current immunization programmes, contributing to the marked reduction in mortality of children less than 5 years of age globally from 93 deaths per 1,000 live births in 1990 to 39 deaths per 1,000 live births in 2018.[2]

Besides preventing 2-3 million deaths per year, vaccination is saving other millions from debilitating consequences from infections. People are living longer and with fewer consequences from the typical problems related to polio, diphtheria, smallpox, and many others, that have made many people blind, paralyzed, and with a

3

lifelong breathing problem, among other debilitating conditions.

Vaccines exist to prevent a problem. They work by entering our body and letting our immune system know what an enemy looks like. It is as someone would come to inform you that at any moment a criminal may break-in. A vaccine will show a picture of this criminal. This "picture" can be in the form of an attenuated virus or bacteria. In the most modern vaccines, it can be a piece of the genetic code that characterizes a particular feature of this "criminal". Your body will then, based on this information, prepare a highly specialized army to fight that specific invader, whenever he shows up. This is how in a nutshell vaccines work.

To most people, there is no doubt that we have a much easier life today because of vaccines. To most people, not to all.

There are over 31 million people who follow anti-vaccine groups on Facebook, with 17 million people subscribing to similar accounts on YouTube.[3]

The anti-vaxxers as we call them have grown a lot in the past, especially due to misinformation spread in social media. And even more during the COVID-19 pandemic.

In another survey, it was found that while eight in 10 people worldwide (79%) said that vaccinations are safe — and nine in 10 said their own children had been inoculated — higher-income pockets in Europe have less confidence in vaccines than lower-income countries in Africa.[4]

This is easy to understand since most people today in rich countries have not experienced the debilitating effects of the many diseases that they have been vaccinated against or live in an area where most people are vaccinated and therefore are at a much lower risk to get infected. If a person never saw a child (or many) debilitated due to polio or smallpox it is hard for this person to understand the importance of vaccination. They are victims of their own success.

The anti-vaccine movement is not new. It started a long time ago together with the vaccines.

The picture below from James Gillray, a British caricaturist, portraits a criticism against the pocken vaccine from 1802.

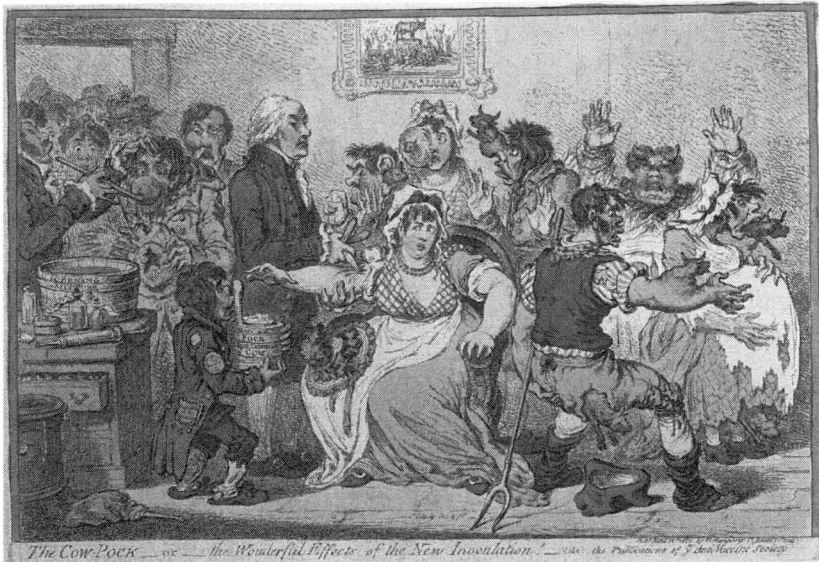

The Cow-Pock __ or __ the Wonderful Effects of the New Inoculation! __ vide. the Publications of ye Anti-Vaccine Society

As you can see above, the picture tries to scare people by making them believe that parts of cows will grow in the bodies of those who are vaccinated.

This sort of misleading and fake news continues ever since. For example, during the COVID-19 pandemic, hundreds of videos, audios and texts were shared via social media trying to scare everyone by claiming that the mRNA-based vaccine would change the DNA of the ones who were vaccinated. Although mRNA vaccines have been tested for decades against cancer and so far, not a single case of a patient with a changed DNA has appeared, the fear is, however, still there.

Another common conspiracy theory is that the promoters of vaccination are trying to reduce the world population. This theory is famous among those who believe AIDS is caused by vaccines, not by the HIV virus.[5] This sort of conspiracy theory is also not new. The American author Eleanor McBean (1905-1989) wrote many books blaming vaccines for all types of problems, including cancer and as the cause for the Spanish flu (1918).[6]

If vaccine promoters were trying to reduce the population by inoculation, they "failed" miserably, since the world population went from 1.8 billion in 1918 to 7.8 billion in 2020, although almost 90% of all children in the world are vaccinated.

The claims we read today against vaccines are nothing, but the recycling of old and wrong ideas.

Below you can see the major claims against vaccines (from anti-vaxxers) according to an interesting research from C. Meyer and S. Reiter from the Robert Koch-Institut in Berlin. [7]

Vaccinations are unnecessary

• The epidemic course of infectious diseases is self-limiting.

• Just improving hygiene and living standards has led to a decrease in infectious diseases.

• There is no proof of the existence of viruses.

• The pathogens do not cause any disease.

• Vaccinations are ineffective because vaccinated people get sick.

Vaccinations are harmful

• They overwhelm, stress, and weaken the immune system.

• They are responsible for the occurrence or increase of other diseases, including chronic ones (including AIDS, autism, diabetes, cancer, multiple sclerosis, sudden infant death syndrome, etc.).

• People who are vaccinated are more likely to get sick or die than those who are not.

• They deprive the organism of the chance to naturally deal with the disease.

• The natural confrontation promotes personal development.

• Immunity after vaccination is lower than after illness.

• The preservatives contained in vaccinations damage the organism.

• Reactivation of the most diverse diseases through live vaccinations is possible.

• The manufacture of vaccines produces contaminants that are responsible for diseases such as BSE and AIDS.

• Vaccinations disrupt the "healthy unity of the individual".

• Viral vaccines change the genetic makeup.

• The overall benefit of vaccinations has not been established. Vaccinations do not reduce the overall burden of damage to health.

• The proportionality of benefit and harm has not been proven.

Vaccinations serve other interests

• They are driven solely by the interests of the pharmaceutical industry.

• They are used against those who think differently.

The purpose of this short book is to debunk one of the most famous fallacies from anti-vaxxers: "Vaccines don't work!", by answering the question "Do vaccines work?"

I'll publish other texts debunking other claims such as "vaccines cause autism" and "it is all about money!"

Therefore, my focus here is to disprove a common belief among anti-vaxxers that vaccines don't work or that they are unnecessary.

How to do it? There is an interesting study showing that empathy instead of data will be more effective to convince anti-vaxxers of the benefit of vaccines.[8]

I could fill the pages of this book with pictures of children suffering from smallpox such as this:

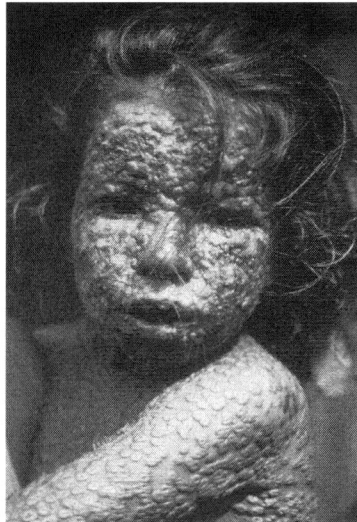

https://en.wikipedia.org/wiki/Smallpox

(Child with smallpox in Bangladesh in 1973)

I could also ask the readers to watch this video below, where a famous skateboarder from Brazil, Og de Souza talks about his paralysis caused by poliomyelitis.

https://www.youtube.com/watch?v=qNWtdYNCK Ms

However, as a scientist, I must use data, science, and logical thinking to make myself understood instead of just sharing sad stories and pictures of people who got sick because they missed immunization. Thus, I decided to use a slightly different method, still based on data and science. As you may have heard or read, most anti-vaxxers won't accept official data, as they claim, "you can't trust the government!" Anti-vaxxers only trust governmental or scientific sources when the data support their views.

Therefore, my only option is to look at the anti-vaxxer's own data and compare it with historical documents and let you and they see where the truth is.

A good friend of mine who is against vaccines has sent some "official" graphics from the anti-vax literature to convince me that vaccines don't work at all.

These graphics will form the base for my discussion throughout this book.

The graphics below show that the numbers of deaths or cases due to infectious diseases were already low when the vaccines were introduced and therefore the population was made to believe the vaccines were the benefactors, when in fact "vaccines did nothing!" As the anti-vaxxers like to claim.

Let's get started on this interesting topic. I must tell you that it was a lot of work, but also a lot of fun to dive into historical documents and see how amazing the development of vaccines has been. Join me now on this ride.

The graphics below are extracted from the presentations and books from Hans U. P. Tolzin, a German journalist and well-known anti-vaxxer who wrote many books against vaccines. He is the owner of Tolzin Publisher.

Chapter 1 - Diphtheria in Germany

The first graphic I looked at is shown below and depicts the number of diphtheria-related deaths in the German territory between 1906 and 1933.

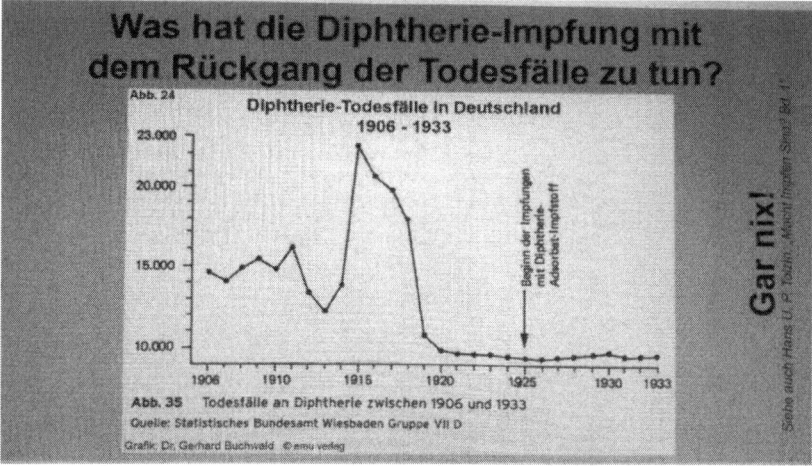

The title of the graphic says: "What does Diphtheria vaccine have to do with the reduction of the number of deaths?" An arrow points to the year 1925 when vaccination started in Germany. On the right side, it is written "Nothing" (Gar nix!) as the answer to the question. Under "Gar nix!" is the reference to the work of Tolzin, the famous German anti-vaxxer.

Let's look at the graphic. Please ignore the increase in the number of deaths between 1914 and 1919. It was the time of World War I. It was chaos in Germany.

As you can see the numbers were already bottom low around 1920, not different from the numbers after the introduction of the vaccine in 1925.

I personally checked the German databases and Indeed the number of death cases is correct and in principle, anyone could think that it is true that vaccination against diphtheria had nothing to do with the elimination of this problem in the German territory... until you dig deeper! I started reading about diphtheria and became amazed by the history behind the development of a vaccine against this serious problem.

Diphtheria is an infection caused by the bacterium *Corynebacterium diphtheriae*[9].

Typical symptoms are a sore throat and fever and potentially developing in severe cases, a grey or white patch in the throat. This can block the airway and create a barking cough as in croup[10]. The neck may swell in part due to enlarged lymph nodes[11]. A form of diphtheria that involves the skin, eyes, or genitals also exists[11,10]. Complications may include myocarditis, inflammation of nerves, kidney, and bleeding problems due to low levels of platelets[11].

14

Myocarditis may result in an abnormal heart rate and inflammation of the nerves may result in paralysis[11].

In 1613, Spain experienced an epidemic of diphtheria. The year is known as *El Año de los Garrotillos* (The Year of Strangulations) in the history of Spain[12].

In 1878, Queen Victoria's daughter Princess Alice and her family became infected with diphtheria, causing two deaths, Princess Marie of Hesse and Rhine and Princess Alice herself[13].

Diphtheria was the number one reason for the death of children between three and five years old in the Prussian region of the German territory in the 19th century.

The authorities wanted a solution, and an incredible group of scientists was brought together:

• Paul Ehrlich
https://en.wikipedia.org/wiki/Paul_Ehrlich

• Shibasaburo Kitasato
https://en.wikipedia.org/wiki/Kitasato_Shibasabur%C5%8D

• Richard Pfeiffer
https://en.wikipedia.org/wiki/Richard_Friedrich_Johannes_Pfeiffer

- August von Wassermann
https://en.wikipedia.org/wiki/August_von_Wasser mann

- Emil von Behring
https://en.wikipedia.org/wiki/Emil_von_Behring
who became the NAME in this case!

In 1890 von Behring and Kitasato immunized guinea pigs with heat-treated diphtheria toxin and published a very short paper (2 pages!) "About the creation of diphtheria immunity and tetanus immunity in animals", this paper not only showed the discovery of the antitoxin in the blood of sick animals, but also a novel immunization method for the treatment of infectious diseases was discovered.

Through animal experiments, they were able to identify that the blood serum of sick animals contained the solution. On November 23th, 1890, von Behring wrote in his laboratory diary: "Is the blood of immune animals able to neutralize the poisonous effect? Yes!"[14] A new era in medicine was about to start!

In only four years they went from discovery to industrial production of the diphtheria healing serum! Next time someone tells you that the COVID-19 vaccine was developed too fast, just tell this person that in the 19th century these scientists took only four years without computers or any of the modern equipment and fast communication we have access to today.

This incredible group of scientists started treating people already in 1894 with the "Behring's Gold", as they named the serum, saving thousands of people right from the beginning. The following year experienced a drastic reduction in the number of cases and continued reducing as they expanded immunization over the years.

In 1901 von Behring won the Nobel prize for medicine and almost every day he received letters from parents thanking him for saving their children! Behring's Gold became the standard to treat diphtheria.

Roughly twenty years later the French Veterinarian Gaston Ramon:

https://en.wikipedia.org/wiki/Gaston_Ramon

turned Behring's concept into the easier form of the vaccine we know today.

Diphtheria is no longer the scary thing it was one-day thanks to a medication (Behring's Gold) that became the first version of the vaccine of today!

Back to the anti-vax graphic. No wonder the diphtheria death cases were already dropping before the vaccine from Gaston Ramon was officially introduced in 1925 because the authorities in Germany were already using a "vaccine" (Behring's Gold) since 1894! If it wouldn't be for this early inoculation program started by the Prussians, Germany wouldn't have saved so many lives before Gaston Ramon came with a better version of a vaccine.

I don't want to start another discussion about this now, but I can't resist making the comment against another typical claim from anti-vaxxers: "Vaccines are dangerous!" If they are dangerous and caused the problem they were supposed to treat (as many claims!) How come the number of infected people didn't increase dramatically after 1925? Immunization was made more available using a new version of a vaccine. If vaccines were the problem, we were supposed to see an increase in cases! Anyway, I hope this claim is debunked by now!

But just to conclude our discussion on this topic.

In early June 2015, a case of diphtheria was diagnosed at Vall d'Hebron University Hospital in Barcelona, Spain. The 6-year-old child who died of the illness had not been previously vaccinated due to parental opposition to vaccination[15].

It was the first case of diphtheria in the country since 1986 as reported by "El Mundo"[16] or from 1998, as reported by WHO[17].

Below you have a beautiful painting showing the production of Bering's Gold by the extraction of blood from horses.

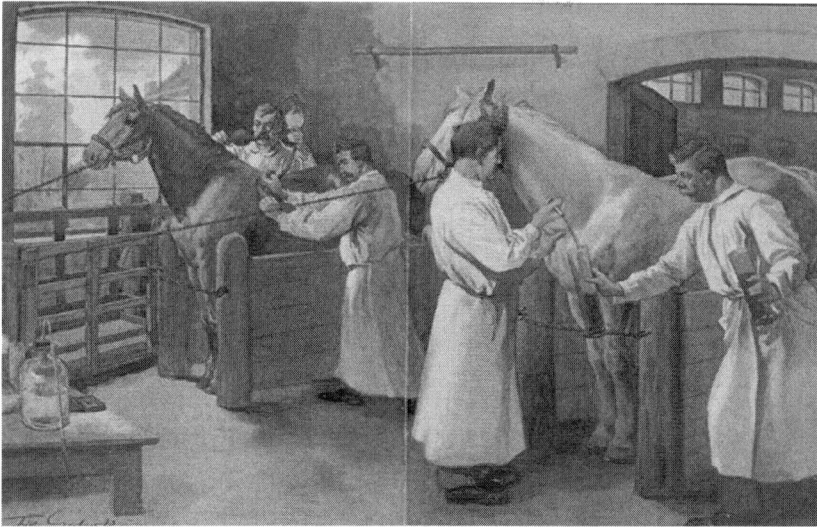

Illustration of the extraction of diphtheria healing serum on horses (Marburg). Fritz Gehrke, 1906. Photos: Philipps University of Marburg

We can only pay great respect and be thankful for the laborious work of everyone who was involved in the discovery and production of this vaccine that has saved millions.

Chapter 2 - Diphtheria in Italy

Somehow like the first graphic (diphtheria in Germany), the graphic below shows that the number of diphtheria cases was already reduced in Italy when the vaccine was made obligatory by 1963.

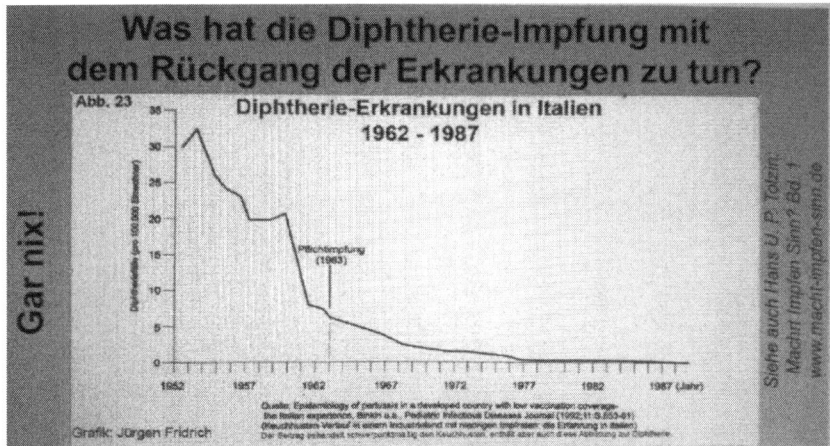

Title of the graphic: "What does the diphtheria vaccine have to do with the reduction in the number of infected people?" On the graphic itself, it is written "Diphtheria diseases in Italy. 1962 - 1987" On the left side, as an answer to the question, we read "Nothing!" (Gar nix!). On the right side, you find the reference from Tolzin, the famous German anti-vaxxer.

What the anti-vaxxers fail to see or say, when talking about this graphic, as in the case of Germany, Italy was already vaccinating its population a long time before! How do I know? I found the information in this remarkably interesting scientific document from Germany:

ERGEBNISSE
DER HYGIENE BAKTERIOLOGIE
IMMUNITÄTSFORSCHUNG UND
EXPERIMENTELLEN
THERAPIE

FORTSETZUNG DES JAHRESBERICHTS
ÜBER DIE ERGEBNISSE DER IMMUNITÄTSFORSCHUNG

UNTER MITWIRKUNG HERVORRAGENDER FACHLEUTE

HERAUSGEGEBEN VON

PROFESSOR DR. WOLFGANG WEICHARDT
WIESBADEN

ELFTER BAND

MIT 32 ZUM TEIL FARBIGEN ABBILDUNGEN

BERLIN
VERLAG VON JULIUS SPRINGER
1930

Translation:

Results of the hygiene-bacteriology immunity research and experimental therapy

22

Continuation of the yearly report about the results
of the immunity research

With the participation of outstanding specialists

Issuing of

Professor Dr. Wolfgang Weichardt

Wiesbaden

Eleventh Volume

With 91 partly colored illustrations

Berlin

Publisher Julius Springer

1930

On page 678 of this document, I found this
important footnote:

[1] Anm.: Dem Vorgehen Frankreichs ist in jüngster Zeit auch Italien gefolgt. In einem Runderlaß vom 21. Okt. 1929 hat die italienische Regierung die Diphtherieschutzimpfung, namentlich mittels Anatoxin aufs wärmste empfohlen. An einer Stelle des Erlasses heißt es z. B.: „Es sollten alle Mittel angewandt werden, um Publikum und Familien von dem großen Segen der Impfung zu überzeugen, die nicht nur die Sterblichkeit der Diphtherie vermindert, sondern auch die gefährlichen Komplikationen und ernsten Folgen der nicht tödlichen Fälle vermeiden hilft". (Vgl. „Die Diphtherieschutzimpfung in Italien" in Il Policlinico vom 13. I. 1930.)

Translation:

Recently, Italy has also followed France's approach. In a circular of October 21, 1929, the Italian government strongly recommended vaccination against diphtheria, namely using anatoxin. At one point of the decree, it says for example: "Every means should be used to convince audiences and families of the great blessing of vaccination, which not only reduces the mortality of diphtheria but also helps avoid the dangerous complications and serious consequences of non-fatal cases". (See "Diphtheria vaccination in Italy" in Il Policlinico of January 13, 1930)

As you can read above the Italian government was already **strongly** recommending **vaccination against diphtheria** before 1930.

Again, no wonder the number of cases was already reduced by 1963 in Italy. The Italian government was already using the vaccine for at least 30 years before it became mandatory! Another evidence that this method was working is the fact that the government made it mandatory.

Today, every government knows that vaccination is one of the best methods to save money in the long run. Having a healthy population leads to a more productive working force and people who financially contribute to the system and fewer people who rely on the government to survive. It is much cheaper to vaccinate than to have a bed in the hospital, medical-material, equipment, and personnel to take care of a sick person.

A study from Johns Hopkins Bloomberg School of Public Health, published in the Health Affairs journal in 2016 says every dollar spent on vaccination saves up to 44 dollars by reducing healthcare spending and productivity loss and curbing the broader economic impact of illness. The study assessed 10 vaccine-preventable infections: *Haemophilus influenzae* type b, hepatitis B, human *papillomavirus*, Japanese encephalitis, measles, *Neisseria meningitis* serogroup A, rotavirus, rubella, *Streptococcus pneumoniae,* and yellow fever[18].

I think we can move to the next graphic!

Chapter 3 - Pertussis vaccine

Whooping cough, also known as pertussis or the 100-day cough, is a highly contagious bacterial disease.

Once again, anti-vaxxers claim (as shown in the picture below) that the vaccine was introduced in the '40s (arrow pointing to year with the word "Impfung" = vaccine) in the USA while the number of pertussis death-related cases was already at an incredibly low number, therefore vaccines are not responsible for the decrease in the number of deaths.

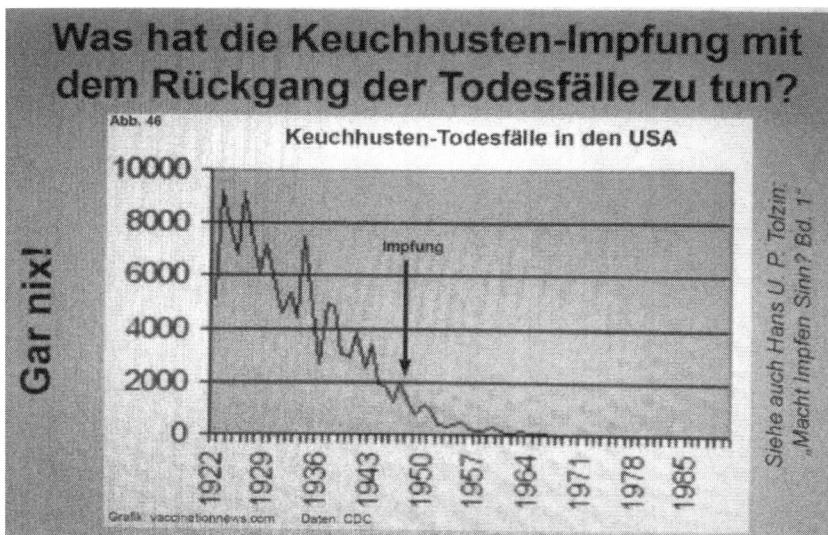

Was hat die Keuchhusten-Impfung mit dem Rückgang der Todesfälle zu tun?

Keuchhusten-Todesfälle in den USA

Title: "What does Pertussis vaccine have to do with the reduction in death cases?" In the white top part of the graphic, it is written "Pertussis death cases in the USA." As an answer to the question, we find "Nothing" (Gar nix!) on the left side and the reference on the right.

Pertussis is caused by the bacterium *Bordetella pertussis*. It is spread easily through the coughs and sneezes of an infected person.

The tendency of pertussis to be milder in adults, sometimes escaping diagnosis, further complicates disease transmission. The coughing associated with the disease may be mild enough in an adult case to be mistaken as a simple cold. The adult, however, will still be contagious and can easily spread the disease to infants too young to be vaccinated, or to individuals whose immunity has waned[19].

The first recorded description of a pertussis epidemic was made by a Parisian, Guillaume de Baillou, in 1578.[20] Read below how graphic his description of the disease is:

"The lung is so irritated by every attempt to expel that which is causing the trouble it neither admits the air nor again easily expels it. The patient is seen to swell up and as if strangled holds his breath tightly in the middle of his throat . . . For they are without the troublesome coughing for the space of four or five hours at a time, then this paroxysm of coughing returns, now so severe that blood is expelled with force through the nose and the mouth. Most frequently an upset stomach follows. . . . For we have seen so many coughing in such a manner, in whom after a vain attempt semi putrid matter in an incredible quantity was ejected."

Nobody knows exactly why pertussis was not described before de Baillou's description. W. H. Holmes[20] attributed the lack of a prior description to an earlier preoccupation of physicians with other serious infections such as plague, smallpox, and typhus and to the possibility that they may have relegated the care of pertussis patients to "old women."[21]

An estimated 16.3 million people worldwide were infected in 2015.[22] Most cases occur in the developing world, and people of all ages may be affected.[23, 24] In 2015, pertussis resulted in 58,700 deaths – down from 138,000 deaths in 1990.[25,26] The bacterium that causes the infection was discovered in 1906.[25] The pertussis vaccine became available in the 1940s.

There are still open questions related to pertussis. For example, the incidence rates of pertussis are consistently higher in females than they are in males across all geographic areas and ages, except for children less than age 1 year.[21] The excess of cases in females, which has been evident in both the pre-and post-vaccination eras, differs from other communicable diseases of childhood, which tend to occur more frequently in males.[27, 28]

Mortality rates, like incidence rates, are highest in the first 6 months of life. The case fatality rate for infants less than age 6 months has been reported to be 0.5 percent.[42] Case fatality rates, like attack rates, are reported to be higher in females than in males. The reasons for this are not clear.[29]

In the earliest decades of the 20th century, infection with *Bordetella pertussis* was essentially universal by school entry. A high cumulative incidence and roughly 1 death per 10 cases meant that pertussis killed more children in the United States annually than polio and measles combined.[30]

Pertussis was made notifiable in the United States in 1922. For 2 decades, reported cases were never under 100,000 and in 1934 peaked at over 265,000.[30] Results of a clinical trial documenting the effectiveness of a killed, whole-cell vaccine became available in 1940 and shortly after the vaccine became available. In 1943 the American Academy of Pediatrics suggested routine use of whole-cell pertussis vaccine, and in 1948 reported cases of pertussis in the United States dropped below 100,000 for the first time. historic low of disease—1010 cases—was recorded in 1976. See the picture below from an awesome paper from T. A. Clark.[30]

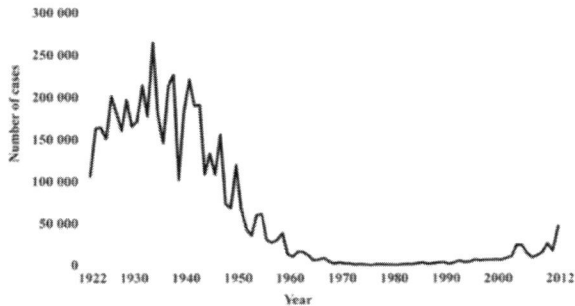

Pertussis cases by year – United States, 1922–2012. Source: Centers for Disease Control and Prevention, National Notifiable Diseases Surveillance System and Supplemental Pertussis Surveillance System and 1922–1949 passive reports to the US Public Health Service.

Now please, compare both graphics. This one (number of cases per year) with the first one (number of deaths per year) used by anti-vaxxers to claim that vaccines don't do anything.

If you look at the year 1940 you will see that the number of cases was still very large, over

200,000 cases, similar to the years before (except for one peak 265,000 in 1934).

What happened after the vaccine was introduced? A clear drop in the number of infections! This is exactly what a vaccine must do: to reduce the infection rate!

The anti-vaxxers look at the drop in the number of deaths and try to persuade others that since the deaths were reducing before the vaccine, then inoculation was not doing anything or not necessary! One has to look at the infection rate to understand the value of a vaccine!

But how to explain the reduction in the number of deaths before the vaccine? I'll answer this question with one word: **antibiotics!**

As Clark[30] shows in his article, pertussis was made notifiable in the United States in 1922. People were dying, but doctors didn't know what to do to save them, moreover, antibiotics would still take 6 years to be discovered (1928). Because it is caused by a bacterium, patients can also be treated with antibiotics. Even today antibiotics may be given to individuals in contact with the patient to prevent infection.

It means before a vaccine could be used, doctors were treating the patients, reducing the number of deaths and of course, if you heal someone, you reduce the probability this person will contaminate someone else. But the real reduction in infection came with the vaccine!

It is also important to notice that when a disease is new to a location, doctors will struggle initially until they find the best method to treat a patient. The same phenomenon was observed with COVID-19; doctors didn't know exactly what to do at the beginning of the 2020 pandemic, therefore many lives were lost during treatment especially in the beginning. The treatment success rate improved overtime after a series of experimental methods and drugs were tested. But only the arrival of a vaccine would reduce the infection rate considerably.

Another common argument used by anti-vaxxers to prove that vaccines don't work is the fact that even after the introduction of a vaccine, vaccinated people may get sick or the resurgence of the disease takes place. The anti-vax groups present such news as if scientists deny or try to cover them up. This is far from the truth. Such issues are closely observed and investigated and made public. More recently this issue was discussed again because of a resurgence of pertussis on two occasions in the US. The causes of these two transitions in pertussis epidemiology remain hotly debated, though their findings suggest that evolution of the *Bordetella pertussis* bacterium, loss of immunity, and persistent transmission among adults, and demographic drivers are more probable explanations for this issue.[31]

Concerning this recent resurgence of pertussis, other scientists have suggested that there is no re-emergence per se, but that increased awareness of pertussis by physicians, especially in adolescents and adults, coupled with improved laboratory methods for its detection, have resulted in reduced under-reporting and a more accurate picture of *B. pertussis* circulation in the population.[32, 33]

In other words, scientists are aware of this issue and that we need to improve both treatments and prevention (vaccination).

With the development and widespread use of effective pertussis vaccines, dramatic changes were affected in the epidemiology of pertussis. However, the recent resurgence in many countries should prompt a closer look at the aspects of pertussis that cause it to persist.[30] In other words, the scientific world doesn't close its eyes to the problem. We all know, we still don't have a perfect solution, but vaccination is much better than non-vaccination!

What however concerns me the most is the fact that anti-vaxxers would rather treat than prevent pertussis. They think it is better to get sick (with all the risks associated with it) than avoiding the disease in the first place by employing vaccination. Because they think that treating with antibiotics is less risky than a vaccine!

Although it is a fact that antibiotics have decreased the number of deaths, it doesn't mean it is the best option in the long run. For the following reasons:

1.   Vaccinated people have less severe cases of pertussis. A study between 2010 and 2012 conducted enhanced Pertussis surveillance for 1.7 million residents in the Portland, Oregon metropolitan area.[34] What have they observed? Vaccinated cases of pertussis had decreased morbidity characterized by less severe illness and significantly reduced illness duration.

2.   Bacteria can develop resistance and therefore we may create a much bigger problem later if we decide to treat instead of preventing the occurrence of pertussis.[9]

3.   And even scarier is the fact that Infants younger than six months of age are particularly at risk for complications and death from pertussis. Complications include pneumonia (bacterial or viral), seizures, ear infections, and dehydration, among others; in adults, rib fracture from

coughing is also possible. The most common of these complications in infants is *B. pertussis* pneumonia, which accompanies almost all deaths from pertussis.[35]

A clear indication of the importance of vaccination is evidenced by the fact that the incidence of the disease increased substantially in those countries that had stopped their vaccination programs, resulting in high levels of morbidity and mortality.[36]

Another indicating factor that vaccination works is that since the mid-twentieth century, global efforts to control/eradicate pertussis began by implementing widespread immunization programs.[37, 38] Before immunization programs were in place, the typical time interval between outbreaks of pertussis was every 2 to 3 years which increased to 3 to 4 years following the implementation of comprehensive vaccination programs.[39, 40]

Because of the complexity of this disease, the vaccines used until now don't offer long-life protection. The following paragraph was extracted from a particularly good article from Nicole Guiso[41]:

https://www.ncbi.nlm.nih.gov/pmc/articles/PMC3967663/

"*B. pertussis*, the agent of the disease, is a small Gram-negative bacterium of the genus *Bordetella*. It is a strict human pathogen. Other members of the genus *Bordetella*, in particular *B. parapertussis*, may cause pertussis-like disease. Unlike in the case of *Corynebacterium diphteriae*, it was difficult to identify the agent of the disease, and indeed, its isolation took 6 years and the development of a complicated medium. This is an important point that many scientists now, more than a century later, forget: it is very difficult to isolate and grow the bacterium reproducibly. Again, unlike *C. diphtheriae*, it was not possible to characterize its toxin(s) rapidly, and consequently, the first vaccine developed was a pertussis whole cell (Pw) vaccine, i.e. a vaccine composed of heat-killed bacteria. It took about 70 years to develop an acellular vaccine, that is a vaccine containing only detoxified bacterial proteins."

He continues in another part of his paper: "Another epidemiological change was associated with a modification of the transmission of the disease which was observed 30 years after the introduction of vaccination of young children. There was an increase in the number of infants admitted to the hospital due to contact with infected older siblings or infected parents. Thus, the child-to-child transmission was replaced by adolescent/adult-to-infant transmission. These observations led to several transmission studies in developed countries, which showed that neither vaccine-induced nor natural immunity is lifelong and that whooping cough can affect individuals of all ages. This disease is not exclusively pediatric."

What does it mean? It means we still must develop better vaccines. We have a long way to go, but what we have achieved so far has been amazing!

Without any doubt, we can affirm that non-vaccinated children will be more likely to have the disease and suffer from neurologic complications such as seizures and encephalopathy, otitis media, anorexia, and dehydration. Complications resulting from pressure effects of severe paroxysms include pneumothorax, epistaxis, subdural hematomas, hernias, and rectal prolapse.[42]

After all this discussion it is important to remember that anti-vaxxers still believe natural immunity should be enough to save us from infections, therefore, they believe, there is no need for vaccines. I wish they could tell this story to the 90% of the pre-Columbian populations of the Americas, who died because of viruses and bacteria that were spread when the first Europeans started to sneeze in the American continent. Common vaccine-preventable diseases killed more native Indians than the colonizers' swords and guns. For more on this topic, please refer to the interesting work of Nielsen "A Disability History of the United States.[43]"

Chapter 4 - HPV vaccine

Cervical cancer usually develops slowly over time. Before cancer appears in the cervix, the cells of the cervix go through changes known as dysplasia, in which abnormal cells begin to appear in the cervical tissue. Over time, the abnormal cells may become cancer cells and start to grow and spread more deeply into the cervix and to surrounding areas.[44]

Risk factors for cervical cancer include the following[45]:

•   Being infected with human papillomavirus (HPV). This is the most important risk factor for cervical cancer.

•   Being exposed to the drug DES (diethylstilbestrol) while in the mother's womb.

•   In women who are infected with HPV, the following risk factors add to the increased risk of cervical cancer:

> ▪ Giving birth to many children.
>
> ▪ Smoking cigarettes.
>
> ▪ Using oral contraceptives ("the Pill") for a long time.

There are also risk factors that increase the risk of HPV infection:

- Having a weakened immune system caused by immunosuppression. Immunosuppression weakens the body's ability to fight infections and other diseases. The body's ability to fight HPV infection may be lowered by long-term immunosuppression from:

  - Being infected with the human immunodeficiency virus (HIV).
  - Taking medicine to help prevent organ rejection after a transplant.
  - Being sexually active at a young age.
  - Having many sexual partners.

Human papillomavirus infection (HPV) causes more than 90% of cases.[46, 47]

More than 500,000 women are diagnosed with cervical cancer each year and over 300,000 dies from it, according to the World Health Organization.[48]

Anti-vaxxers claim that the HPV vaccine is doing nothing against HPV-related cancers. For this, the anti-vaxxers around the world, especially the ones in Germany, make use of this graphic below.

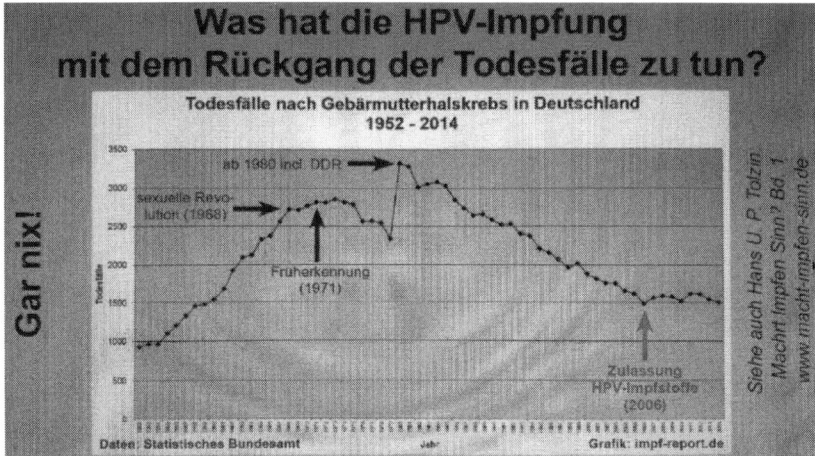

Title of the graphic: "What does the HPV vaccine have to do with the reduction of death cases?" In the white part (right on the top of the graphic) it is written "Death cases due to cervical cancer in Germany 1952 - 2014". On the graphic itself it is written "sexual revolution (1968)", "early detection (1971)", "from 1980 included DDR (East Germany)", "Approval of HPV-vaccine (2006)". On the left side, the common quote from all graphics "Nothing!" (Gar nix!) is the answer to the question, and on the right side the famous reference.

As we can see in the graphic above, the purpose is to show that the death rate due to cervical cancer (mostly caused by HPV) was already low enough when the vaccine was introduced (after 2006) and there was no change in the death rate and therefore, the new vaccine was doing nothing!

Again, as in some of the graphics before, the focus is the death rate, not the infection rate. Based on what we learned so far, you can guess what will come next, right? Yes, the people who use this graphic to try to prove vaccines are not working, just miss again the most important role of a vaccine. Vaccines exist to avoid infections and consequently reduce the potential outcomes of such infections (among them death). However, I don't believe that anyone on earth would find that getting cancer is an option, as long as the treatment can save him or her!

Most people know that cancer diagnosis and treatment have improved a lot in the past years, which means patients get diagnosed earlier and get a higher success rate from cancer treatment.

As long as medical science advances, we are supposed to see a decrease in the number of deaths, because we have access to better treatments. And this is exactly what we see in this graphic! In 1971 early detection became a major tool to fight this type of cancer, which was growing dramatically in numbers as you can see in the graphic before 1971. The earlier someone starts a cancer treatment the better. However, every single cancer therapy has strong side effects. In some cases, they can be devastating!

What the graphic shows us is that we found better ways of avoiding a patient's death, but we were not preventing an infection. The person who got infected will most likely survive, after going through cancer treatment! Just in case you don't know, there is no "nice" cancer treatment as well as there is no guarantee a patient will survive.

The most important point that this graphic above misses completely is the following statement from an interesting article from Buttmann-Schweiger et al.[49]: "in Germany, HPV vaccination commenced in 2007 for 12–17-year-old girls. As the oldest vaccinated women from the birth cohort of 1990 will not reach age 35 until 2023, it will be 2038 before the 35–49 age-group consists entirely of potentially vaccinated women."

In case you didn't understand, the results of the vaccination that started in 2007 will mostly be seen decades later, for a very obvious reason, HPV-related cancers develop slowly.

It is estimated that a total of 120,000 new cancer cases in men and women in more developed countries could be avoided if exposure to HPV was prevented.[50]

But we can already appreciate the effectiveness of this vaccination program to prevent this disease. A research, published in *The Lancet in 2019*, analyzed the health outcomes of 66 million people under 30 in 14 high-income countries, including Germany. It showed that, in countries where the vaccine had been given out for more than five years, there was an 83% reduction in two strains of HPV in 15- to 19-year-old girls and a 66% reduction in women aged 20 to 24.[51]

Boys and men were also shown to have benefitted; anal and genital warts reduced by half among teenage boys and by a third for those between 20 to 24. Warts also dropped by 67% among teenage girls, 54% among women aged 20 to 24, and 31% in women aged 25 to 29.[51]

As the HPV vaccine has only been available for just over 10 years, it's too soon to measure how these programmes might impact rates of cervical cancer itself, but the results so far are very promising.[52]

Conclusion & lessons for today

Anti-vaccine is not new, but unfortunately, a big movement, mostly fed by exaggeration, misinterpretation, fear, and fake news associated with all sorts of conspiracy theories. Such theories and claims are also not new but mostly recycled from old urban legends or conspiracy theories that can be traced back to 100 or even 200 years ago. The anti-vax movement is not based on science, but on confirmation bias and a strong desire to believe that vaccines are among the evil things invented by some individuals holding hidden agendas.

During the COVID-19 pandemic it was almost impossible not to be confronted every single day with fake news: "Bill Gates wanted to implant a chip in humans by means of a vaccine", "vaccines cause DNA change", "the government wants to reduce the world population", and many others. Besides such allegations, we were also bombarded with misinterpretation of data.

During a debate on the internet where I was invited to explain how the new mRNA-based vaccines work, someone challenged me with an interesting piece of information: "the death rate in Mozambique due to COVID is extremely low. Do we really need a vaccine? Or should we just copy what they are doing?"

45

Such doubts can easily deceive many.

To answer this question, I want you to look at the following graphic:

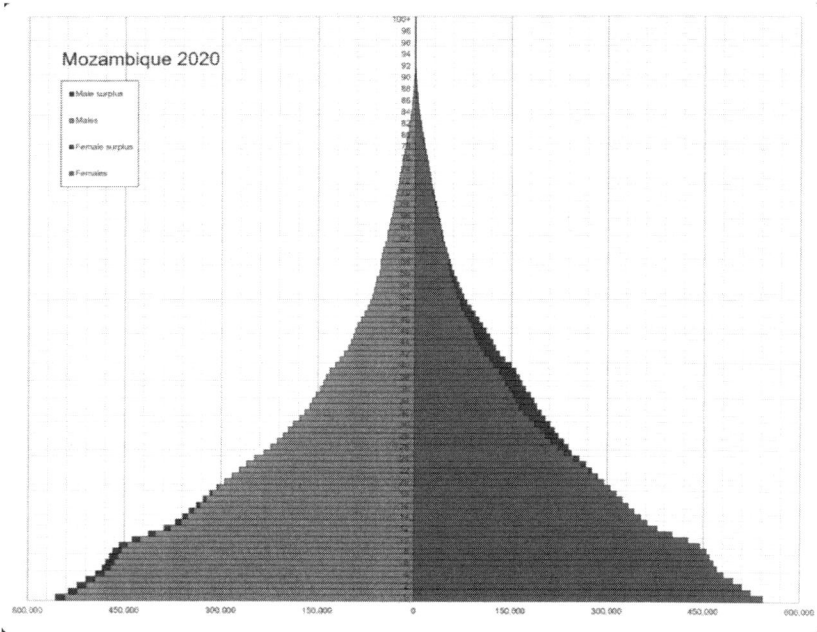

Mozambique 2020

■ Male surplus
■ Males
■ Female surplus
■ Females

This is the demographic distribution of the population in Mozambique. At the bottom of the graphic, it is possible to see a large population of children and young people. As you climb the graphic finding the older age groups, you can see a drastic reduction in the number of people. This indicates that, because of many factors such as malnutrition, bad infrastructure and inadequate access to basic healthcare, the population in Mozambique dies at an early age. The life expectancy of Mozambique is unfortunately only of 54.1 years.

As you may know the age group that is the most vulnerable to COVID is exactly the one that we almost don't find in Mozambique, namely people above 75 years old.

The picture below from the CDC compares age groups and risk for infection, hospitalization and death due to COVID-19.[53]

Compared to younger adults, older adults are more likely to require hospitalization if they get COVID-19

Risk for COVID-19 Infection, Hospitalization, and Death By Age Group								
Rate compared to 5-17-years[1]	0-4 years	5-17 years	18-29 years	30-39 years	40-49 years	50-64 years	65-74 years	75-84 years	85+ years
Cases[2]	<1x	Reference group	3x	2x	2x	2x	2x	2x	2x
Hospitalization[3]	2x	Reference group	7x	10x	15x	25x	35x	55x	80x
Death[4]	2x	Reference group	15x	45x	130x	400x	1100x	2800x	7900x

All rates are relative to the 5-17 year age category. Sample interpretation: Compared with 5-17 year olds, the rate of death is 45 times higher in 30-39 year olds, and 7,900 times higher in 85+ year olds. Compared with 18-29 year olds, the rate of hospitalization is 8 times higher in 75-84 year olds (55 divided by 7 equals 7.9).

Just as a comparison, see below the demographics of the UK, where one can easily spot a large elderly population. The population that is mostly vulnerable to COVID-19.

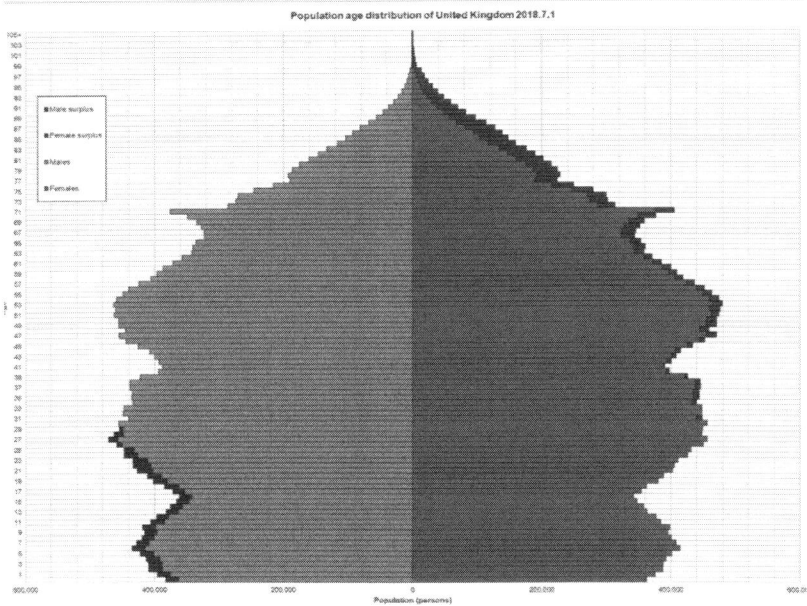

Population age distribution of United Kingdom 2018.7.1

Such age distribution is typical for developed countries. Therefore, it is not a surprise that developed countries had on average higher death rate than others with low life expectancy.

Moreover, Mozambique is among the countries with the lowest number of daily COVID-19 tests per thousand people. These two factors combined will give us a clear idea why we find a low death rate due to COVID-19 in Mozambique.

This simple example can teach us how to deal with news and even more important with fake news!

Another sort of ridiculous news I had to listen to almost daily during COVID-19, was that "we shouldn't wear masks, because they are dangerous!" In 1920 the USA and Germany approved a new guideline for surgeries[54], where all surgeons and nurses had to wear masks during such procedures. It means that in the last 100 years, these professionals have been wearing masks every day, but there is not a single study indicating that they have a shorter life span than ordinary people, who don't wear masks.

Most anti-vaxxers come from rich countries, where immunization programs have been in place for decades, therefore they never saw children suffering from poliomyelitis or hospitals filled with children coughing to death or struggling with smallpox or about to die because of other vaccine-preventable diseases. They are victims of their own success!

As I said in the beginning, most supporters of anti-vax groups won't accept official data that clearly indicate the effectiveness of vaccines, but for those who are still open to read scientific papers and learn from data, please see below this amazing table published in 2007 at the Journal of

American Medical Association. You can download the original paper here[56]:

https://jamanetwork.com/journals/jama/fullarticle/209448

As you can see above, for all vaccine-preventable diseases, there was a drastic reduction in the number of cases and deaths. The last two columns show the reduction in the percentage of the number of cases and deaths (values in parentheses). In most cases, the reduction is close or equal to 100%!

It came as no surprise that the anti-vax movement have been trying as much as possible to downplay the need and the potential effectiveness of COVID-19 vaccines. But now we can see the infection rate dropping as Israel's vaccination program is approaching 50% of its population.

A recent study has shown that "the vaccine was equally effective in all age groups and became the most effective one week after the second vaccination. Furthermore, data from Israel show that Covid-19 hospitalizations have been declining in the vaccinated age groups, while in groups that have not yet received the vaccine, hospitalization remains unchanged."[55]

I hope it is clear by now that vaccines work! They are not yet perfect, but nothing in this world is. Therefore, millions of dollars are invested every year in the development of better vaccines. But as discussed in this book, we are in incredibly good hands with the vaccines we have available at this moment. We should appreciate that.

References

1.   World Health Organization. Global vaccine action plan 2011–2020. *WHO* https://www.who.int/immunization/global_vaccine_action_plan/GVAP_doc_2011_2020/en/ (2013).

2.   World Health Organization. Child mortality and causes of death. WHO https://www.who.int/gho/child_health/mortality/mortality_under_five_text/en/ (2020).

3.   https://www.thelancet.com/journals/landig/article/PIIS2589-7500(20)30227-2/fulltext

4.   https://www.marketwatch.com/story/this-is-the-most-anti-vaxxer-country-in-the-world-2019-06-19

5.   https://en.wikipedia.org/wiki/HIV/AIDS_denialism

6.   https://www.psiram.com/en/index.php?title=Eleanor_McBean&mobileaction=toggle_view_mobile

7.   Meyer C and Reite S. Impfgegner und Impfskeptiker: Geschichte, Hintergründe, Thesen, Umgang Article in Bundesgesundheitsblatt - Gesundheitsforschung - Gesundheitsschutz · Bundesgesundheitsbl - Gesundheitsforsch -

Gesundheitsschutz 2004 · 47:1182–1188 DOI
10.1007/s00103-004-0953-x.

8.   https://today.duke.edu/2020/12/convince-
vaccine-skeptics-use-empathy-information-and-
re-start-experts-say

9.   Atkinson, W (May 2012). Diphtheria
Epidemiology and Prevention of Vaccine-
Preventable Diseases (12 ed.). Public Health
Foundation. pp. 215–230. ISBN 9780983263135.

10.   "Diphtheria vaccine". Wkly Epidemiol Rec.
81 (3): 24–32. 20 January 2006. PMID 16671240.

11.   Atkinson, W (May 2012). Diphtheria
Epidemiology and Prevention of Vaccine-
Preventable Diseases (12 ed.). Public Health
Foundation. pp. 215–230. ISBN 9780983263135.

12.   Laval, Enrique (March 2006). "El garotillo
(Difteria) en España (Siglos XVI y XVII)". Revista
Chilena de Infectología. 23 (1): 78–80.

13.   https://www.alexanderpalace.org/palace/ali
cehessebio.php

14.   https://www.aerzteblatt.de/archiv/173215/
125-Jahre-Diphtherieheilserum-Das-Behring-
sche-Gold

15.   "Parents of diphtheria-stricken boy feel
"tricked" by anti-vaccination groups". El Pais. 5
June 2015. Archived.
https://web.archive.org/web/20150607000140/ht

tp://elpais.com/elpais/2015/06/05/inenglish/1433
512717_575817.html

16.   "Primer caso de difteria en España en casi
30 años". *El Mundo*. 2 June 2015.
http://www.elmundo.es/salud/2015/06/02/556db
c3d268e3e16598b4589.html

17.   "WHO – Diphtheria reported cases".
http://apps.who.int/immunization_monitoring/glo
balsummary/timeseries/tsincidencediphtheria.htm
l

18.   https://www.vaccinestoday.eu/stories/vacc
ines-save-lives-and-money/

19.   https://www.historyofvaccines.org/content/
articles/pertussis-whooping-cough

20.   Holmes WH. Bacillary and rickettsial
infections: acute and chronic: a textbook. Black
death to white plague. New York: Macmillan;
1940.

21.   Howson CP, Howe CJ, Fineberg HV, editors.
Institute of Medicine (US) Committee to Review
the Adverse Consequences of Pertussis and
Rubella Vaccines; Howson CP, Washington (DC):
National Academies Press (US); 1991.

22.   Vos, Theo; Allen, Christine; Arora, Megha;
Barber, Ryan M.; Bhutta, Zulfiqar A.; Brown,
Alexandria; Carter, Austin; Casey, Daniel C.;
Charlson, Fiona J.; Chen, Alan Z.; Coggeshall,
Megan; Cornaby, Leslie; Dandona, Lalit; Dicker,

Daniel J.; Dilegge, Tina; Erskine, Holly E.; Ferrari, Alize J.; Fitzmaurice, Christina; Fleming, Tom; Forouzanfar, Mohammad H.; Fullman, Nancy; Gething, Peter W.; Goldberg, Ellen M.; Graetz, Nicholas; Haagsma, Juanita A.; Hay, Simon I.; Johnson, Catherine O.; Kassebaum, Nicholas J.; Kawashima, Toana; et al. (October 2016). "Global, regional, and national incidence, prevalence, and years lived with disability for 310 diseases and injuries, 1990–2015: a systematic analysis for the Global Burden of Disease Study 2015". Lancet. 388 (10053): 1545–1602.

23.   Heininger U (February 2010). "Update on pertussis in children". Expert Review of Anti-Infective Therapy. 8 (2): 163–73

24.   Wang K, Bettiol S, Thompson MJ, Roberts NW, Perera R, Heneghan CJ, Harnden A (September 2014). "Symptomatic treatment of the cough in whooping cough". The Cochrane Database of Systematic Reviews. 9 (9): CD003257.

25.   Wang, Haidong; Naghavi, Mohsen; Allen, Christine; Barber, Ryan M.; Bhutta, Zulfiqar A.; Carter, Austin; Casey, Daniel C.; Charlson, Fiona J.; Chen, Alan Zian; Coates, Matthew M.; Coggeshall, Megan; Dandona, Lalit; Dicker, Daniel J.; Erskine, Holly E.; Ferrari, Alize J.; Fitzmaurice, Christina; Foreman, Kyle; Forouzanfar, Mohammad H.; Fraser, Maya S.; Fullman, Nancy;

Gething, Peter W.; Goldberg, Ellen M.; Graetz, Nicholas; Haagsma, Juanita A.; Hay, Simon I.; Huynh, Chantal; Johnson, Catherine O.; Kassebaum, Nicholas J.; Kinfu, Yohannes; et al. (October 2016). "Global, regional, and national life expectancy, all-cause mortality, and cause-specific mortality for 249 causes of death, 1980–2015: a systematic analysis for the Global Burden of Disease Study 2015". Lancet. 388 (10053): 1459–1544.

26.   GBD 2013 Mortality Causes of Death Collaborators (January 2015). "Global, regional, and national age-sex specific all-cause and cause-specific mortality for 240 causes of death, 1990–2013: a systematic analysis for the Global Burden of Disease Study 2013". Lancet. 385 (9963): 117–71

27.   Cherry JD. 1984. The epidemiology of pertussis and pertussis immunization in the United Kingdom and the United States: a comparative study. Current Problems in Pediatrics 14:1-78.

28.   Gordon JE, Hood RI. 1951. Whooping cough and its epidemiological anomalies. American Journal of Medical Science 222:333-361.

29.   Cherry JD, Brunell PA, Golden GS, Karzon DT. 1988. Report of the task force on pertussis

and pertussis immunization—1988. Pediatrics 81(6, part 2):939-984.

30.   Clark, TA. Changing Pertussis Epidemiology: Everything Old is New Again. The Journal of Infectious Diseases, Volume 209, Issue 7, 1 April 2014, Pages 978–981, https://doi.org/10.1093/infdis/jiu001

31.   Rohani P and Draked JM. The decline and resurgence of pertussis in the US. Epidemics 3: 183–188 (2011)

32.   Cherry, J., 2003. The science and fiction of the "resurgence" of pertussis. Pediatrics 112, 405.

33.   Cherry, J.D., 2005. The epidemiology of pertussis: a comparison of the epidemiology of the disease pertussis with the epidemiology of Bordetella pertussis infection. Pediatrics 115, 1422–1427.

34.   https://web.archive.org/web/20150301120 339/http://cid.oxfordjournals.org/content/early/2 014/03/14/cid.ciu156.abstract

35.   https://www.historyofvaccines.org/content/ articles/pertussis-whooping-cough

36.   Zepp F, Heininger U, Mertsola J, et al. Rationale for pertussis booster vaccination throughout life in Europe. Lancet Infect Dis 2011;11(7):557-70.

37.   Jackson D, Rohani P. Perplexities of pertussis: recent global epidemiological trends and their potential causes. Epidemiol Infect 2014;142(4):672-84.

38.   de Greeff SC, Dekkers AL, Teunis P, et al. Seasonal patterns in time series of pertussis. Epidemiol Infect 2009;137(10):1388-95.

39.   Ghorbani GR, Zahraei SM, Moosazadeh M, et al. Comparing seasonal pattern of laboratory confirmed cases of pertussis with clinically suspected cases. Osong Public Health Res Perspect 2016;7(2):131-7.

40.   Broutin H, Guégan J-F, Elguero E, et al. Large-scale comparative analysis of pertussis population dynamics: periodicity, synchrony, and impact of vaccination. Am J Epidemiol 2005;161(12):1159-67.

41.   Guiso, N. How to fight pertussis? Ther Adv Vaccines. 1(2) 59–66 DOI: 10.1177/2051013613481348 (2013).

42.   https://www.cdc.gov/vaccines/pubs/pinkbook/downloads/pert.pdf

43.   Nielsen, K.E. (2012). A Disability History of the United States. Beacon Press. ISBN 9780807022047.

44.   https://www.aacr.org/patients-caregivers/cancer/cervical-cancer/#:~:text=Cervical%20cancer%20usually

%20develops%20slowly,appear%20in%20the%2
0cervical%20tissue.

45.   https://www.cancer.gov/types/cervical/pati
ent/cervical-treatment-pdq#section/all

46.   Kumar V, Abbas AK, Fausto N, Mitchell RN
(2007). *Robbins Basic Pathology* (8th ed.).
Saunders Elsevier. pp. 718–721. ISBN 978-1-
4160-2973-1.

47.   Kufe, Donald (2009). *Holland-Frei cancer
medicine* (8th ed.). New York: McGraw-Hill
Medical. p. 1299. ISBN 9781607950141.

48.   https://www.dw.com/en/tried-and-true-
hpv-vaccination-shows-sharp-drop-in-cancer-
causing-infections/a-49398419

49.   Buttmann-Schweiger, N., Deleré, Y., Klug,
S.J. et al. Cancer incidence in Germany
attributable to human papillomavirus in 2013.
BMC Cancer 17, 682 (2017).
https://doi.org/10.1186/s12885-017-3678-6

50.   de Martel C, Ferlay J, Franceschi S, Vignat J,
Bray F, Forman D, Plummer M. Global burden of
cancers attributable to infections in 2008: a
review and synthetic analysis. Lancet Oncol.
2012;13(6):607–15.

51.   Drolet M, Bénard É, Pérez N, Brisson M,
HPV. Population-level impact and herd effects
following the introduction of human
papillomavirus vaccination programmes: updated

systematic review and meta-analysis. Lancet. 394(10197):497. (2019).

52.   https://www.dw.com/en/tried-and-true-hpv-vaccination-shows-sharp-drop-in-cancer-causing-infections/a-49398419

53.   https://www.cdc.gov/coronavirus/2019-ncov/need-extra-precautions/older-adults.html#:~:text=The%20greatest%20risk%20for%20severe,intensive%20care%2C%20or%20a

54.   https://www.ncbi.nlm.nih.gov/pmc/articles/PMC7309199/pdf/40001_2020_Article_423.pdf

55.   https://www.pharmaceutical-technology.com/comment/israel-covid-19-cases/

56.   Roush et al. Historical Comparisons of Morbidity and Mortality for Vaccine-Preventable Diseases in the United States. Vol 298, No. 18: 2155-2163 (2007)

https://jamanetwork.com/journals/jama/fullarticle/209448

Printed in Great Britain
by Amazon

85696036R00036